This Medical Journal Belongs To:

This journal is an organization tool used at your own risk. It is not intended to be a medical treatment or provide medical suggestions. It should not be used in place of standard medical care by a licensed medical doctor.

MEDICAL HISTORY

NAME:

BIRTH DATE:

ALLERGIES:

BLOOD TYPE:

FAMILY DOCTOR:

CONTACT:

MEDICATIONS:

DATE:	SURGERIES, MAJOR EVENTS, ETC	NOTES:

FAMILY MEDICAL OVERVIEW

HEALTH INSURANCE INFORMATION

DENTAL INSURANCE INFORMATION

OTHER INSURANCE INFORMATION

OTHER INSURANCE INFORMATION

IMPORTANT INFORMATION

ALLERGIES

WHAT:　　　　　　**WHO:**

BLOOD TYPES

NAME:　　　　　　**BLOOD TYPE:**

IMMUNIZATIONS

NAME:

DATE:	TYPE:	PURPOSE:	DOCTOR:

SURGERY DETAILS

NAME: **DATE:**

DATE:	TYPE OF SURGERY & REASON:	DOCTOR:	HOSPITAL:

THE FIRST YEAR

FAMILY DOCTORS

FAMILY DOCTOR
- NAME:
- ADDRESS:
- PHONE:
- ADDITIONAL INFORMATION:

FAMILY DENTIST
- NAME:
- ADDRESS:
- PHONE:
- ADDITIONAL INFORMATION:

OPTOMETRIST
- NAME:
- ADDRESS:
- PHONE:
- ADDITIONAL INFORMATION:

PEDIATRICIAN
- NAME:
- ADDRESS:
- PHONE:
- ADDITIONAL INFORMATION:

DENTIST
- NAME:
- ADDRESS:
- PHONE:
- ADDITIONAL INFORMATION:

SPECIALTY DOCTORS

ONCOLOGIST

NAME:

ADDRESS:

PHONE:

ADDITIONAL INFORMATION:

NAME:

ADDRESS:

PHONE:

ADDITIONAL INFORMATION:

NAME:

ADDRESS:

PHONE:

ADDITIONAL INFORMATION:

NAME:

ADDRESS:

PHONE:

ADDITIONAL INFORMATION:

NAME:

ADDRESS:

PHONE:

ADDITIONAL INFORMATION:

ADDITIONAL CONTACTS

NAME:	NAME:	NAME:
PHONE:	PHONE:	PHONE:
EMAIL:	EMAIL:	EMAIL:
ADDRESS:	ADDRESS:	ADDRESS:

NAME:	NAME:	NAME:
PHONE:	PHONE:	PHONE:
EMAIL:	EMAIL:	EMAIL:
ADDRESS:	ADDRESS:	ADDRESS:

NAME:	NAME:	NAME:
PHONE:	PHONE:	PHONE:
EMAIL:	EMAIL:	EMAIL:
ADDRESS:	ADDRESS:	ADDRESS:

NOTES:

MEDICAL CHECKUPS

MONTH:	MONTH:	MONTH:
MONTH:	MONTH:	MONTH:
MONTH:	MONTH:	MONTH:

BLOOD PRESSURE

DATE:	TIME:	BLOOD PRESSURE:	PULSE:

DIETITIAN RECOMMENDATIONS

As of Date:_____

MEAL PLAN

EXERCISE

NOTES

BLOOD SUGAR TRACKER

	BEFORE		MEALS	1 HR	2 HRS	3 HRS
MONDAY		B L D S				
TUESDAY		B L D S				
WEDNESDAY		B L D S				
THURSDAY		B L D S				
FRIDAY		B L D S				

Use only if instructed to monitor blood sugar by a doctor

BLOOD SUGAR TRACKER

	BEFORE		MEALS	1 HR	2 HRS	3 HRS
SATURDAY		B				
		L				
		D				
		S				
SUNDAY		B				
		L				
		D				
		S				

NOTES

Use only if instructed to monitor blood sugar by a doctor

MEDICATIONS

NAME: **MONTH:**

MEDICATION:	USED FOR:	DOSE:	TIMES PER DAY:

SCANS & IMAGING

NAME:

DATE:	TYPE:	PURPOSE:	RESULTS:

BLOOD TESTS

NAME:

DATE:	TYPE:	DOCTOR:	RESULTS:

HOSPITAL VISITS

NAME:

DATE:	REASON FOR VISIT OR STAY:	HOSPITAL/ DOCTOR:	DISCHARGE DATE:

DOCTOR VISITS

NAME:

DATE:	DOCTOR:	REASON:	RESULTS:

EXAM TRACKER

NAME:	DATE:	DOCTOR:	REASON:	NEXT APPT:

NAME:	DATE:	DOCTOR:	REASON:	NEXT APPT:

NAME:	DATE:	DOCTOR:	REASON:	NEXT APPT:

NAME:	DATE:	DOCTOR:	REASON:	NEXT APPT:

ILLNESS TRACKER

DATE:	DESCRIPTION:	DR. VISIT	TREATMENT
		☐	☐
		☐	☐
		☐	☐
		☐	☐
		☐	☐
		☐	☐
		☐	☐
		☐	☐
		☐	☐
		☐	☐
		☐	☐
		☐	☐
		☐	☐
		☐	☐
		☐	☐
		☐	☐
		☐	☐
		☐	☐
		☐	☐
		☐	☐

SYMPTOMS TRACKER

DATE:	DESCRIPTION:	DR. VISIT	TREATMENT
		☐	☐
		☐	☐
		☐	☐
		☐	☐
		☐	☐
		☐	☐
		☐	☐
		☐	☐
		☐	☐
		☐	☐
		☐	☐
		☐	☐
		☐	☐
		☐	☐
		☐	☐
		☐	☐
		☐	☐
		☐	☐
		☐	☐
		☐	☐
		☐	☐

DENTAL VISITS

DENTAL RECORDS FOR:

DENTAL OFFICE:

DATE:	DESCRIPTION:	NEXT APPOINTMENT:

MEDICAL APPOINTMENTS

MEDICAL RECORDS FOR:

DOCTOR OFFICE:

DATE:	DESCRIPTION:	NEXT APPOINTMENT:

DOCTOR VISITS

DATE: **FOLLOW UP:**

DOCTOR:

HOSPITAL:

REASON/PURPOSE:

NOTES:

DATE: **FOLLOW UP:**

DOCTOR:

HOSPITAL:

REASON/PURPOSE:

NOTES:

TEST RESULTS

PERIOD OF:

DATE:	TEST:	DOCTOR:	PURPOSE:	RESULTS

MONTHLY HEALTH TRACKER

JANUARY	FEBRUARY	MARCH

APRIL	MAY	JUNE

MONTHLY HEALTH TRACKER

JULY	AUGUST	SEPTEMBER

OCTOBER	NOVEMBER	DECEMBER

YEARLY HEALTH TRACKER

YEAR: _____

JANUARY	FEBRUARY	MARCH

APRIL	MAY	JUNE

JULY	AUGUST	SEPTEMBER

OCTOBER	NOVEMBER	DECEMBER

NOTES:

MEDICAL EXPENSES

YEAR:

DATE:	DESCRIPTION:	INSURANCE %:	COST:

Notes

THE SECOND YEAR

FAMILY DOCTORS

FAMILY DOCTOR
NAME:
ADDRESS:
PHONE:
ADDITIONAL INFORMATION:

FAMILY DENTIST
NAME:
ADDRESS:
PHONE:
ADDITIONAL INFORMATION:

OPTOMETRIST
NAME:
ADDRESS:
PHONE:
ADDITIONAL INFORMATION:

PEDIATRICIAN
NAME:
ADDRESS:
PHONE:
ADDITIONAL INFORMATION:

DENTIST
NAME:
ADDRESS:
PHONE:
ADDITIONAL INFORMATION:

SPECIALTY DOCTORS

ONCOLOGIST

NAME:

ADDRESS:

PHONE:

ADDITIONAL INFORMATION:

NAME:

ADDRESS:

PHONE:

ADDITIONAL INFORMATION:

NAME:

ADDRESS:

PHONE:

ADDITIONAL INFORMATION:

NAME:

ADDRESS:

PHONE:

ADDITIONAL INFORMATION:

NAME:

ADDRESS:

PHONE:

ADDITIONAL INFORMATION:

ADDITIONAL CONTACTS

NAME:	NAME:	NAME:
PHONE:	PHONE:	PHONE:
EMAIL:	EMAIL:	EMAIL:
ADDRESS:	ADDRESS:	ADDRESS:
NAME:	NAME:	NAME:
PHONE:	PHONE:	PHONE:
EMAIL:	EMAIL:	EMAIL:
ADDRESS:	ADDRESS:	ADDRESS:
NAME:	NAME:	NAME:
PHONE:	PHONE:	PHONE:
EMAIL:	EMAIL:	EMAIL:
ADDRESS:	ADDRESS:	ADDRESS:

NOTES:

MEDICAL CHECKUPS

MONTH:

MONTH:

MONTH:

MONTH:

MONTH:

MONTH:

MONTH:

MONTH:

MONTH:

BLOOD PRESSURE

DATE:	TIME:	BLOOD PRESSURE:	PULSE:

DIETITIAN RECOMMENDATIONS

As of Date:_____

MEAL PLAN

EXERCISE

NOTES

BLOOD SUGAR TRACKER

	BEFORE		MEALS	1 HR	2 HRS	3 HRS
MONDAY		B				
		L				
		D				
		S				
TUESDAY		B				
		L				
		D				
		S				
WEDNESDAY		B				
		L				
		D				
		S				
THURSDAY		B				
		L				
		D				
		S				
FRIDAY		B				
		L				
		D				
		S				

Use only if instructed to monitor blood sugar by a doctor

BLOOD SUGAR TRACKER

	BEFORE		MEALS	1 HR	2 HRS	3 HRS
SATURDAY		B				
		L				
		D				
		S				
SUNDAY		B				
		L				
		D				
		S				

NOTES

Use only if instructed to monitor blood sugar by a doctor

MEDICATIONS

NAME: **MONTH:**

MEDICATION:	USED FOR:	DOSE:	TIMES PER DAY:

SCANS & IMAGING

NAME:

DATE:	**TYPE:**	**PURPOSE:**	**RESULTS:**

BLOOD TESTS

NAME:

DATE:	**TYPE:**	**DOCTOR:**	**RESULTS:**

HOSPITAL VISITS

NAME:

DATE:	REASON FOR VISIT OR STAY:	HOSPITAL/ DOCTOR:	DISCHARGE DATE:

DOCTOR VISITS

NAME:

DATE:	DOCTOR:	REASON:	RESULTS:

EXAM TRACKER

NAME:	DATE:	DOCTOR:	REASON:	NEXT APPT:

NAME:	DATE:	DOCTOR:	REASON:	NEXT APPT:

NAME:	DATE:	DOCTOR:	REASON:	NEXT APPT:

NAME:	DATE:	DOCTOR:	REASON:	NEXT APPT:

ILLNESS TRACKER

DATE:	DESCRIPTION:	DR. VISIT	TREATMENT
		☐	☐
		☐	☐
		☐	☐
		☐	☐
		☐	☐
		☐	☐
		☐	☐
		☐	☐
		☐	☐
		☐	☐
		☐	☐
		☐	☐
		☐	☐
		☐	☐
		☐	☐
		☐	☐
		☐	☐
		☐	☐
		☐	☐
		☐	☐

SYMPTOMS TRACKER

DATE:	DESCRIPTION:	DR. VISIT	TREATMENT
		☐	☐
		☐	☐
		☐	☐
		☐	☐
		☐	☐
		☐	☐
		☐	☐
		☐	☐
		☐	☐
		☐	☐
		☐	☐
		☐	☐
		☐	☐
		☐	☐
		☐	☐
		☐	☐
		☐	☐
		☐	☐
		☐	☐
		☐	☐
		☐	☐
		☐	☐
		☐	☐

DENTAL VISITS

DENTAL RECORDS FOR:

DENTAL OFFICE:

DATE:	DESCRIPTION:	NEXT APPOINTMENT:

MEDICAL APPOINTMENTS

MEDICAL RECORDS FOR:

DOCTOR OFFICE:

DATE:	DESCRIPTION:	NEXT APPOINTMENT:

DOCTOR VISITS

DATE: **FOLLOW UP:**

DOCTOR:

HOSPITAL:

REASON/PURPOSE:

NOTES:

DATE: **FOLLOW UP:**

DOCTOR:

HOSPITAL:

REASON/PURPOSE:

NOTES:

TEST RESULTS

PERIOD OF:

DATE:	TEST:	DOCTOR:	PURPOSE:	RESULTS

MONTHLY HEALTH TRACKER

JANUARY	FEBRUARY	MARCH

APRIL	MAY	JUNE

MONTHLY HEALTH TRACKER

JULY	AUGUST	SEPTEMBER

OCTOBER	NOVEMBER	DECEMBER

YEARLY HEALTH TRACKER

YEAR: _____

JANUARY	FEBRUARY	MARCH

APRIL	MAY	JUNE

JULY	AUGUST	SEPTEMBER

OCTOBER	NOVEMBER	DECEMBER

NOTES:

MEDICAL EXPENSES

YEAR:

DATE:	DESCRIPTION:	INSURANCE %:	COST:

Notes

THE THIRD YEAR

FAMILY DOCTORS

FAMILY DOCTOR
NAME:
ADDRESS:
PHONE:
ADDITIONAL INFORMATION:

FAMILY DENTIST
NAME:
ADDRESS:
PHONE:
ADDITIONAL INFORMATION:

OPTOMETRIST
NAME:
ADDRESS:
PHONE:
ADDITIONAL INFORMATION:

PEDIATRICIAN
NAME:
ADDRESS:
PHONE:
ADDITIONAL INFORMATION:

DENTIST
NAME:
ADDRESS:
PHONE:
ADDITIONAL INFORMATION:

SPECIALTY DOCTORS

ONCOLOGIST

NAME:

ADDRESS:

PHONE:

ADDITIONAL INFORMATION:

NAME:

ADDRESS:

PHONE:

ADDITIONAL INFORMATION:

NAME:

ADDRESS:

PHONE:

ADDITIONAL INFORMATION:

NAME:

ADDRESS:

PHONE:

ADDITIONAL INFORMATION:

NAME:

ADDRESS:

PHONE:

ADDITIONAL INFORMATION:

ADDITIONAL CONTACTS

NAME:

PHONE:

EMAIL:

ADDRESS:

NAME:

PHONE:

EMAIL:

ADDRESS:

NAME:

PHONE:

EMAIL:

ADDRESS:

NAME:

PHONE:

EMAIL:

ADDRESS:

NAME:

PHONE:

EMAIL:

ADDRESS:

NAME:

PHONE:

EMAIL:

ADDRESS:

NAME:

PHONE:

EMAIL:

ADDRESS:

NAME:

PHONE:

EMAIL:

ADDRESS:

NAME:

PHONE:

EMAIL:

ADDRESS:

NOTES:

MEDICAL CHECKUPS

MONTH:

MONTH:

MONTH:

MONTH:

MONTH:

MONTH:

MONTH:

MONTH:

MONTH:

BLOOD PRESSURE

DATE:	TIME:	BLOOD PRESSURE:	PULSE:

DIETITIAN RECOMMENDATIONS

As of Date:_____

MEAL PLAN

EXERCISE

NOTES

BLOOD SUGAR TRACKER

	BEFORE		MEALS	1 HR	2 HRS	3 HRS
MONDAY		B				
		L				
		D				
		S				
TUESDAY		B				
		L				
		D				
		S				
WEDNESDAY		B				
		L				
		D				
		S				
THURSDAY		B				
		L				
		D				
		S				
FRIDAY		B				
		L				
		D				
		S				

Use only if instructed to monitor blood sugar by a doctor

BLOOD SUGAR TRACKER

	BEFORE		MEALS	1 HR	2 HRS	3 HRS
SATURDAY		B				
		L				
		D				
		S				
SUNDAY		B				
		L				
		D				
		S				

NOTES

Use only if instructed to monitor blood sugar by a doctor

MEDICATIONS

NAME: **MONTH:**

MEDICATION:	USED FOR:	DOSE:	TIMES PER DAY:

SCANS & IMAGING

NAME:

DATE:	TYPE:	PURPOSE:	RESULTS:

BLOOD TESTS

NAME:

DATE:	TYPE:	DOCTOR:	RESULTS:

HOSPITAL VISITS

NAME:

DATE:	REASON FOR VISIT OR STAY:	HOSPITAL/ DOCTOR:	DISCHARGE DATE:

DOCTOR VISITS

NAME:

DATE:	**DOCTOR:**	**REASON:**	**RESULTS:**

EXAM TRACKER

NAME:	DATE:	DOCTOR:	REASON:	NEXT APPT:

NAME:	DATE:	DOCTOR:	REASON:	NEXT APPT:

NAME:	DATE:	DOCTOR:	REASON:	NEXT APPT:

NAME:	DATE:	DOCTOR:	REASON:	NEXT APPT:

ILLNESS TRACKER

DATE:	DESCRIPTION:	DR. VISIT	TREATMENT
		☐	☐
		☐	☐
		☐	☐
		☐	☐
		☐	☐
		☐	☐
		☐	☐
		☐	☐
		☐	☐
		☐	☐
		☐	☐
		☐	☐
		☐	☐
		☐	☐
		☐	☐
		☐	☐
		☐	☐
		☐	☐
		☐	☐
		☐	☐
		☐	☐
		☐	☐

SYMPTOMS TRACKER

DATE:	DESCRIPTION:	DR. VISIT	TREATMENT
		☐	☐
		☐	☐
		☐	☐
		☐	☐
		☐	☐
		☐	☐
		☐	☐
		☐	☐
		☐	☐
		☐	☐
		☐	☐
		☐	☐
		☐	☐
		☐	☐
		☐	☐
		☐	☐
		☐	☐
		☐	☐
		☐	☐
		☐	☐

DENTAL VISITS

DENTAL RECORDS FOR:

DENTAL OFFICE:

DATE:	DESCRIPTION:	NEXT APPOINTMENT:

MEDICAL APPOINTMENTS

MEDICAL RECORDS FOR:

DOCTOR OFFICE:

DATE:	DESCRIPTION:	NEXT APPOINTMENT:

DOCTOR VISITS

DATE: **FOLLOW UP:**

DOCTOR:

HOSPITAL:

REASON/PURPOSE:

NOTES:

DATE: **FOLLOW UP:**

DOCTOR:

HOSPITAL:

REASON/PURPOSE:

NOTES:

TEST RESULTS

PERIOD OF:

DATE:	TEST:	DOCTOR:	PURPOSE:	RESULTS

MONTHLY HEALTH TRACKER

JANUARY	FEBRUARY	MARCH

APRIL	MAY	JUNE

MONTHLY HEALTH TRACKER

JULY	AUGUST	SEPTEMBER

OCTOBER	NOVEMBER	DECEMBER

YEARLY HEALTH TRACKER

YEAR: _____

JANUARY

FEBRUARY

MARCH

APRIL

MAY

JUNE

JULY

AUGUST

SEPTEMBER

OCTOBER

NOVEMBER

DECEMBER

NOTES:

MEDICAL EXPENSES

YEAR:

DATE:	DESCRIPTION:	INSURANCE %:	COST:

Notes

THE FOURTH YEAR

FAMILY DOCTORS

FAMILY DOCTOR
- NAME:
- ADDRESS:
- PHONE:
- ADDITIONAL INFORMATION:

FAMILY DENTIST
- NAME:
- ADDRESS:
- PHONE:
- ADDITIONAL INFORMATION:

OPTOMETRIST
- NAME:
- ADDRESS:
- PHONE:
- ADDITIONAL INFORMATION:

PEDIATRICIAN
- NAME:
- ADDRESS:
- PHONE:
- ADDITIONAL INFORMATION:

DENTIST
- NAME:
- ADDRESS:
- PHONE:
- ADDITIONAL INFORMATION:

SPECIALTY DOCTORS

ONCOLOGIST

NAME:

ADDRESS:

PHONE:

ADDITIONAL INFORMATION:

NAME:

ADDRESS:

PHONE:

ADDITIONAL INFORMATION:

NAME:

ADDRESS:

PHONE:

ADDITIONAL INFORMATION:

NAME:

ADDRESS:

PHONE:

ADDITIONAL INFORMATION:

NAME:

ADDRESS:

PHONE:

ADDITIONAL INFORMATION:

ADDITIONAL CONTACTS

NAME:	NAME:	NAME:
PHONE:	PHONE:	PHONE:
EMAIL:	EMAIL:	EMAIL:
ADDRESS:	ADDRESS:	ADDRESS:

NAME:	NAME:	NAME:
PHONE:	PHONE:	PHONE:
EMAIL:	EMAIL:	EMAIL:
ADDRESS:	ADDRESS:	ADDRESS:

NAME:	NAME:	NAME:
PHONE:	PHONE:	PHONE:
EMAIL:	EMAIL:	EMAIL:
ADDRESS:	ADDRESS:	ADDRESS:

NOTES:

MEDICAL CHECKUPS

☐ MONTH: ☐ MONTH: ☐ MONTH:

☐ MONTH: ☐ MONTH: ☐ MONTH:

☐ MONTH: ☐ MONTH: ☐ MONTH:

BLOOD PRESSURE

DATE:	TIME:	BLOOD PRESSURE:	PULSE:

DIETITIAN RECOMMENDATIONS

As of Date:_____

MEAL PLAN

EXERCISE

NOTES

BLOOD SUGAR TRACKER

	BEFORE		MEALS	1 HR	2 HRS	3 HRS
MONDAY		B				
		L				
		D				
		S				
TUESDAY		B				
		L				
		D				
		S				
WEDNESDAY		B				
		L				
		D				
		S				
THURSDAY		B				
		L				
		D				
		S				
FRIDAY		B				
		L				
		D				
		S				

Use only if instructed to monitor blood sugar by a doctor

BLOOD SUGAR TRACKER

	BEFORE		MEALS	1 HR	2 HRS	3 HRS
SATURDAY		B				
		L				
		D				
		S				
SUNDAY		B				
		L				
		D				
		S				

NOTES

Use only if instructed to monitor blood sugar by a doctor

MEDICATIONS

NAME: **MONTH:**

MEDICATION:	USED FOR:	DOSE:	TIMES PER DAY:

SCANS & IMAGING

NAME:

DATE:	TYPE:	PURPOSE:	RESULTS:

BLOOD TESTS

NAME:

DATE:	**TYPE:**	**DOCTOR:**	**RESULTS:**

HOSPITAL VISITS

NAME:

DATE:	**REASON FOR VISIT OR STAY:**	**HOSPITAL/ DOCTOR:**	**DISCHARGE DATE:**

DOCTOR VISITS

NAME:

DATE:	DOCTOR:	REASON:	RESULTS:

EXAM TRACKER

NAME:	DATE:	DOCTOR:	REASON:	NEXT APPT:

NAME:	DATE:	DOCTOR:	REASON:	NEXT APPT:

NAME:	DATE:	DOCTOR:	REASON:	NEXT APPT:

NAME:	DATE:	DOCTOR:	REASON:	NEXT APPT:

ILLNESS TRACKER

DATE:	DESCRIPTION:	DR. VISIT	TREATMENT
		☐	☐
		☐	☐
		☐	☐
		☐	☐
		☐	☐
		☐	☐
		☐	☐
		☐	☐
		☐	☐
		☐	☐
		☐	☐
		☐	☐
		☐	☐
		☐	☐
		☐	☐
		☐	☐
		☐	☐
		☐	☐
		☐	☐
		☐	☐
		☐	☐

SYMPTOMS TRACKER

DATE:	DESCRIPTION:	DR. VISIT	TREATMENT
		☐	☐
		☐	☐
		☐	☐
		☐	☐
		☐	☐
		☐	☐
		☐	☐
		☐	☐
		☐	☐
		☐	☐
		☐	☐
		☐	☐
		☐	☐
		☐	☐
		☐	☐
		☐	☐
		☐	☐
		☐	☐
		☐	☐
		☐	☐

DENTAL VISITS

DENTAL RECORDS FOR:

DENTAL OFFICE:

DATE:	DESCRIPTION:	NEXT APPOINTMENT:

MEDICAL APPOINTMENTS

MEDICAL RECORDS FOR:

DOCTOR OFFICE:

DATE:	DESCRIPTION:	NEXT APPOINTMENT:

DOCTOR VISITS

DATE: **FOLLOW UP:**

DOCTOR:

HOSPITAL:

REASON/PURPOSE:

NOTES:

DATE: **FOLLOW UP:**

DOCTOR:

HOSPITAL:

REASON/PURPOSE:

NOTES:

TEST RESULTS

PERIOD OF:

DATE:	TEST:	DOCTOR:	PURPOSE:	RESULTS

MONTHLY HEALTH TRACKER

JANUARY	FEBRUARY	MARCH

APRIL	MAY	JUNE

MONTHLY HEALTH TRACKER

JULY	AUGUST	SEPTEMBER

OCTOBER	NOVEMBER	DECEMBER

YEARLY HEALTH TRACKER

YEAR: _____

JANUARY	FEBRUARY	MARCH

APRIL	MAY	JUNE

JULY	AUGUST	SEPTEMBER

OCTOBER	NOVEMBER	DECEMBER

NOTES:

MEDICAL EXPENSES

YEAR:

DATE:	DESCRIPTION:	INSURANCE %:	COST:

Notes

THE FIFTH YEAR

FAMILY DOCTORS

FAMILY DOCTOR
NAME:
ADDRESS:
PHONE:
ADDITIONAL INFORMATION:

FAMILY DENTIST
NAME:
ADDRESS:
PHONE:
ADDITIONAL INFORMATION:

OPTOMETRIST
NAME:
ADDRESS:
PHONE:
ADDITIONAL INFORMATION:

PEDIATRICIAN
NAME:
ADDRESS:
PHONE:
ADDITIONAL INFORMATION:

DENTIST
NAME:
ADDRESS:
PHONE:
ADDITIONAL INFORMATION:

SPECIALTY DOCTORS

ONCOLOGIST

NAME:

ADDRESS:

PHONE:

ADDITIONAL INFORMATION:

NAME:

ADDRESS:

PHONE:

ADDITIONAL INFORMATION:

NAME:

ADDRESS:

PHONE:

ADDITIONAL INFORMATION:

NAME:

ADDRESS:

PHONE:

ADDITIONAL INFORMATION:

NAME:

ADDRESS:

PHONE:

ADDITIONAL INFORMATION:

ADDITIONAL CONTACTS

NAME:

PHONE:

EMAIL:

ADDRESS:

NAME:

PHONE:

EMAIL:

ADDRESS:

NAME:

PHONE:

EMAIL:

ADDRESS:

NAME:

PHONE:

EMAIL:

ADDRESS:

NAME:

PHONE:

EMAIL:

ADDRESS:

NAME:

PHONE:

EMAIL:

ADDRESS:

NAME:

PHONE:

EMAIL:

ADDRESS:

NAME:

PHONE:

EMAIL:

ADDRESS:

NAME:

PHONE:

EMAIL:

ADDRESS:

NOTES:

MEDICAL CHECKUPS

☐ MONTH: ☐ MONTH: ☐ MONTH:

☐ MONTH: ☐ MONTH: ☐ MONTH:

☐ MONTH: ☐ MONTH: ☐ MONTH:

DIETITIAN RECOMMENDATIONS

As of Date:_____

MEAL PLAN

EXERCISE

NOTES

BLOOD PRESSURE

DATE:	TIME:	BLOOD PRESSURE:	PULSE:

BLOOD SUGAR TRACKER

	BEFORE		MEALS	1 HR	2 HRS	3 HRS
MONDAY		B				
		L				
		D				
		S				
TUESDAY		B				
		L				
		D				
		S				
WEDNESDAY		B				
		L				
		D				
		S				
THURSDAY		B				
		L				
		D				
		S				
FRIDAY		B				
		L				
		D				
		S				

Use only if instructed to monitor blood sugar by a doctor

BLOOD SUGAR TRACKER

	BEFORE		MEALS	1 HR	2 HRS	3 HRS
SATURDAY		B				
		L				
		D				
		S				
SUNDAY		B				
		L				
		D				
		S				

NOTES

Use only if instructed to monitor blood sugar by a doctor

MEDICATIONS

NAME: **MONTH:**

MEDICATION:	USED FOR:	DOSE:	TIMES PER DAY:

SCANS & IMAGING

NAME:

DATE:	TYPE:	PURPOSE:	RESULTS:

BLOOD TESTS

NAME:

DATE:	TYPE:	DOCTOR:	RESULTS:

HOSPITAL VISITS

NAME:

DATE:	REASON FOR VISIT OR STAY:	HOSPITAL/ DOCTOR:	DISCHARGE DATE:

DOCTOR VISITS

NAME:

DATE:	**DOCTOR:**	**REASON:**	**RESULTS:**

EXAM TRACKER

NAME:	DATE:	DOCTOR:	REASON:	NEXT APPT:

NAME:	DATE:	DOCTOR:	REASON:	NEXT APPT:

NAME:	DATE:	DOCTOR:	REASON:	NEXT APPT:

NAME:	DATE:	DOCTOR:	REASON:	NEXT APPT:

ILLNESS TRACKER

DATE:	DESCRIPTION:	DR. VISIT	TREATMENT
		☐	☐
		☐	☐
		☐	☐
		☐	☐
		☐	☐
		☐	☐
		☐	☐
		☐	☐
		☐	☐
		☐	☐
		☐	☐
		☐	☐
		☐	☐
		☐	☐
		☐	☐
		☐	☐
		☐	☐
		☐	☐
		☐	☐
		☐	☐
		☐	☐

SYMPTOMS TRACKER

DATE:	DESCRIPTION:	DR. VISIT	TREATMENT
		☐	☐
		☐	☐
		☐	☐
		☐	☐
		☐	☐
		☐	☐
		☐	☐
		☐	☐
		☐	☐
		☐	☐
		☐	☐
		☐	☐
		☐	☐
		☐	☐
		☐	☐
		☐	☐
		☐	☐
		☐	☐
		☐	☐
		☐	☐
		☐	☐
		☐	☐
		☐	☐
		☐	☐

DENTAL VISITS

DENTAL RECORDS FOR:

DENTAL OFFICE:

DATE:	DESCRIPTION:	NEXT APPOINTMENT:

MEDICAL APPOINTMENTS

MEDICAL RECORDS FOR:

DOCTOR OFFICE:

DATE:	DESCRIPTION:	NEXT APPOINTMENT:

DOCTOR VISITS

DATE:

DOCTOR:

HOSPITAL:

REASON/PURPOSE:

NOTES:

FOLLOW UP:

DATE:

DOCTOR:

HOSPITAL:

REASON/PURPOSE:

NOTES:

FOLLOW UP:

TEST RESULTS

PERIOD OF:

DATE:	TEST:	DOCTOR:	PURPOSE:	RESULTS

MONTHLY HEALTH TRACKER

JANUARY	FEBRUARY	MARCH

APRIL	MAY	JUNE

MONTHLY HEALTH TRACKER

JULY	AUGUST	SEPTEMBER

OCTOBER	NOVEMBER	DECEMBER

YEARLY HEALTH TRACKER

YEAR: _____

JANUARY

FEBRUARY

MARCH

APRIL

MAY

JUNE

JULY

AUGUST

SEPTEMBER

OCTOBER

NOVEMBER

DECEMBER

NOTES:

MEDICAL EXPENSES

YEAR:

DATE:	DESCRIPTION:	INSURANCE %:	COST:

Notes

Notes

Notes

www.ingramcontent.com/pod-product-compliance
Lightning Source LLC
Chambersburg PA
CBHW081002170526
45158CB00010B/2872